DEDICATION

This book is dedicated to my dear husband Joseph. If it were not for his love and support I probably would not be alive today. He got me out of my state of depression about my weight and helped me to get healthy.

Unconditional love and support can move mountains.

TABLE OF CONTENTS

CHAPTER 1- WHAT IS THE METABOLISM?

Your metabolism is the amount of energy in calories that your body burns in order to maintain its weight. Whether you're sleeping, running, sitting, standing, riding in a car or eating a bowl of chocolate fudge ice cream, your body is constantly burning calories in order to keep you going. Think of it as a fire within you, burning your fat and food away. No, sorry but you won't burn enough calories chewing your chocolate fudge ice cream to cancel out the calories you just took in by eating that bowl of ice cream. It would be nice if it worked that way, but it doesn't.

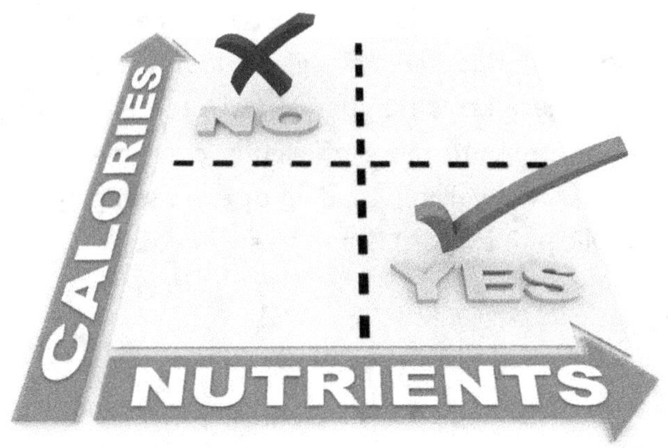

Get any group of women together, and even some men, get them talking on the topic of their metabolism and you'll hear moaning and groaning and complaining about how their metabolism is so slow, that when they were younger they could eat anything they wanted to and not gain weight but now if they simply *think* about a piece of cheesecake they put five pounds on.

It's a sad but true fact of life that as we age our metabolism slows down. It doesn't stop (although at times we might feel as though it has) but it does change. The reason for this is because we have more lean muscle mass at 20 than we do at 70, and lean muscle mass is what helps burn calories.

Some people have higher metabolisms than others and are able to burn off the calories they eat and never gain an ounce. Others have metabolisms slower than a slug and everything they eat seems to stick with them and not get burned off. No two people are alike in the calories they burn and the rate of their metabolism.

Having said that, is it possible to boost your metabolism in order to burn more calories and be able to lose weight? Evidence suggests that there are a number of ways to help maximize our metabolism in order to more efficiently consume the food we eat, whether we're walking, reading or even sleeping. Boosting your metabolic rate is possible and I'll show you how.

Don't Diet

When we see beautiful models in magazines and svelte actresses in movies, we are tempted to cut down on our eating in order to lose weight and look more like them. We decide to stop eating as much so we can drops some pounds. Less food taken in should mean you'll lose weight quickly, right? Not necessarily. Our bodies are very efficient at storing food as fat as a defense against starvation. When you cut your calories, and if you do it drastically enough, your body panics. Think of it in terms of an army and its rations.

Body: "Danger! Danger! There's not enough food! We're starving!"

Metabolism: "Cut down on production men, we're going into survival mode! Slow and steady!

Emphasis on the slow!"

Body: "Just make sure we have enough fat stores to get through this famine"

Metabolism: "Aye Aye Captain!"

Orders have been given and voila', thunder thighs are born. Or Jelly Bellies, saggy arms, double chins, saddle bags and any number of fat stores are created in order to make sure that your body doesn't starve. Think of it as the general of an army, laying in stores for a very long winter. When your body is in survival mode, it takes fewer calories to sustain itself, to maintain its current weight. Excess calories are stored as fat and the stores are parceled out to the soldiers reluctantly and very s l o w l y in order to make sure the resources last as long as possible.

Severe restriction of calories is a sure fire way to cause your metabolism to slow down to a crawl. If you've been crash dieting for years without exercising then your metabolism has been affected. Dieting like this burns muscle and the less muscle mass you have, the less calories you burn and the slower your metabolism. You will now need fewer calories to maintain your current weight. This means that if you consume more calories, your body won't need to use them for energy and will store them. Helloooo belly fat.

When you put the weight back on, and you will if you've been crash dieting, then it will be put back on as fat. This means that your metabolic rate has probably dropped a little bit each time that you've crash dieted. Putting on more fat and losing muscle will cause your metabolism to slow down even more. It seems like a cycle of doom, doesn't i? It can be if you don't break that cycle. I'm about to show you just how to increase your metabolism in order to burn the most calories possible, even when you're sleeping.

CHAPTER 2- BOOSTING THE METABOLISM TAKES WORK

Yes, it's true. If you want to boost your metabolism, the very best thing you can do is to start moving your body. Some exercise is good for building muscle and some is good for just plain sweating and giving you a good cardio workout.

While aerobic exercises like running, jogging, playing tennis or riding a bike will help you tone your body and maintain your weight, they don't do a whole lot to increase your muscle mass- which is what you need to do in order to boost your metabolism.

Weight training and strength training help build muscle tissue and this is a good thing. Think of your body, again, in terms of an army. Too much fat means too many soldiers are weak and wounded, not able to carry on the fight.

Body: "Sir! Our numbers have been depleted! We're not efficiently fighting the incoming calories, I mean missiles!"

Metabolism: "Recruit new soldiers, FRESH soldiers! Put them on the front lines and let them take on the calories! I mean missiles!

Body: "Sir, yes Sir! Commence lifting weights NOW!"

As you increase your muscle mass, and decrease your fat stores, your metabolism speeds up. It burns more of what you eat. Your body will require more calories to maintain itself, so if you increase your soldiers, I mean muscle mass, through weight training and strength training, and consume a lower calorie amount, you will lose weight. Just don't lower your calories so drastically that it sends your army into survival and hoard mode again.

Boosting your metabolism through exercise is just one way to light up those calorie burning fires within you.

Start Eating

Yep. Eat. You have to eat in order to keep your metabolism running in an optimal manner. Are you skipping breakfast in order to cut back on calories and lose weight? Bad battle plan, soldier. Let's work out a battle plan together here and I'll show you just why you need to eat, when you should eat and what you should eat.

Remember that not eating sends your army into survival mode, right? It believes you are starving and so slows down it's metabolism in order to conserve its stores. Let's say you've been asleep for 8 hours. You didn't have anything to eat for two to three or more hours before you went to bed last night. Now your body has been without food for about 11 or 12 hours. If you skip breakfast, you're adding more time and your body is starting to whimper and wonder where its fuel is and if it's ever going to come and should it start conserving now because starvation is just around the corner? You've got your little soldiers all up in a lather and that's not a good thing.

Now, what happens if you go to bed, get up and eat a healthy breakfast? You have, in essence, broken your fast. You've been fasting for ten or more hours and now it's over. Your little soldiers can relax and get back to their normal duty, which is burning calories instead of storing them.

Eat small meals and eat them often during the day. Research has shown that breaking down the traditional three meals a day into six smaller meals, spaced evenly throughout the day will result in a boost to your metabolism.

No this does not mean you can go out and have a meal from a fast food restaurant in the morning, a steak and fries two hours later, five Twinkies and a ho-ho next, then tacos with sour cream and guacamole for your next meal, BBQ ribs with mashed potatoes for your fifth meal and a trip to that all-you-can-stuff-into-yourself-buffet at the mall for your sixth and final meal of the day. Sure, you might be boosting your metabolism a bit, but you're overcompensating with too many calories and losing the Battle of the Bulge in a BIG way. Your soldiers will be so over-run with calories that they will be forced to store them as fat.

Break down your meals into six smaller and HEALTHIER meals during the day. Lower your caloric intake in a healthy manner and your little soldiers will not only win the battle, you've given them the right weapons to win the entire war.

Also, avoid white in your diet. Simple sugars, rice and refined flour are all absorbed quickly by your body and are turned into fat stores. Eat more complex carbohydrates. They take a longer time to be absorbed into your body and this enables your blood sugar to remain level. Try eating brown rice instead of white rice, whole grains in your breads and pasta made from wheat flour instead of white refined flours.

Avoid caffeine and drink green tea instead. Caffeine is known to bock absorption of vitamin C, create a bit of unhealthy acid in your system and stimulate sugar cravings. If there's one thing you don't need when you're trying to lose weight, its sugar cravings. Green tea has antioxidants and doesn't have all those nasty side effects that coffee can give you.

Burn Calories and Lose Weight Now

Drink at least 8 glasses of water a day. Water flushes out all the toxins that are set free when you're losing weight. If you are dehydrated, your metabolism slows down. Try drinking very cold water when you're pushing the H2O. Your body has to remain warm and it will boost your metabolism a bit each time it has to warm up after your glass of ice water.

CHAPTER 3- THE BASICS OF BURNING FAT

If you're overweight, you are not a bad person. You're simply overweight. But it's important to lose the extra pounds so you'll look good, feel healthier and develop a sense of pride and self-esteem. Once you've lost the fat, you'll need to maintain your weight.

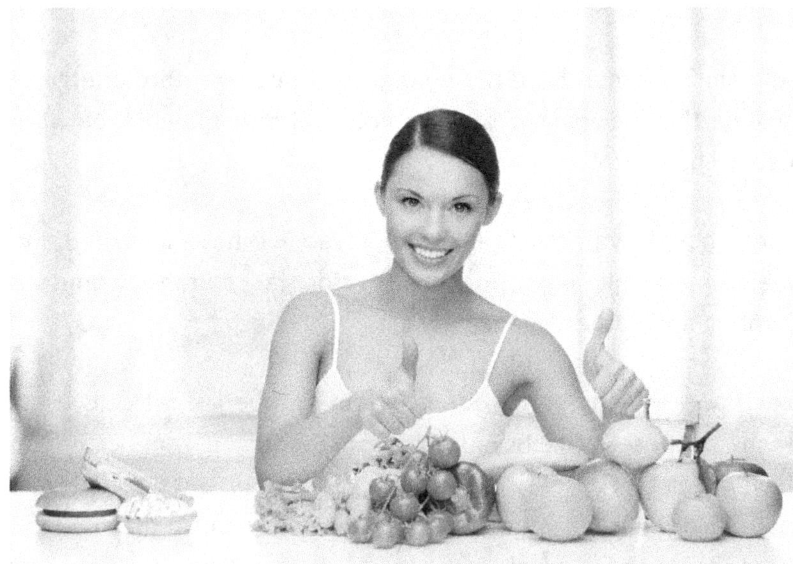

In this booklet, you'll discover how to lose 10 pounds a month – a nice, safe loss of about two or two-and-a-half pounds a week – painlessly. You'll feel satisfied and more energetic than in the past without feeling deprived.

Most Americans pack on those extra pounds by eating the wrong things. Changing these poor eating habits is the key to long-term success. Knowledge – along with the right food – is the key.

When humans lived in caves, they didn't know anything about preserving and storing food. They spent all their waking time and energy hunting and gathering food. When they had it, they gobbled it down fast. Instead of storing food in pantries or cupboards, they stored energy in their bodies in the form of fat to burn during periods when there was little or nothing to eat.

Each year, it was absolutely vital for them to put on a good layer of fat during the warm sprint and summer months. That was the only way they could guarantee their survival during the lean and mean winter months.

And since women bore the young, they needed more energy to sustain themselves and their babies, and that meant they were usually heavier.

Even though we no longer live in caves, we have inherited and maintained this basic mechanism for fat storage from our hunting and gathering ancestors.

Each one of us is born with a certain number of fat cells. How many of these fat cells you possess depends on genetics. If you have a lot of fat cells, maybe your ancestors were the biggest people in the tribe, which was a good thing because they had the best chances of survival.

You can never get rid of fat cells, but – unfortunately – you can add to them. Depending upon what you eat, your body will manufacture new far cells. And like those you were born with, they never go away.

That doesn't mean you're doomed to be fat once you put on extra pounds. It is possible to shrink fat cells. That's what happens when you lose weight. You burn up the fat stored in those big fat cells. Think of them as balloons. Burning off the fat inside them has the same effect as letting the air out of a balloon.

A good weight loss program requires a certain amount of intake restriction – the consumption of fewer calories. You burn off the fat by eating less fat and becoming more active.

To guarantee a lifetime of weight-control success, you have to change the type of foods you eat, so that you ingest less fat and still get the vitamins, minerals, trace elements, protein, fat and carbohydrates your body needs to thrive.

Extremely low-calorie diets may help you shed pounds quickly, but they'll lead to failure in the long run.

That's because humans are genetically protected against starvation. During food shortages, our bodies slow down our metabolisms and burn less energy so we can stay alive.

A part of our brain called the hypothalamus keeps us on an even weight keep by creating a "set point." That's the weight where we feel comfortable. The hypothalamus determines this point based on the level of consumption it's used to. It seeks to keep our weight constant, even if that point is over what it should be.

When we drastically cut back our food intake, the brain thinks the body is starving, and in an effort to preserve life, it slows the metabolism. Soon the pounds stop coming off. Consequently, we grow hungry and uncomfortable and then eat more. And then the diet fails.

How can you compensate for this metabolic slow-down? The answer is that you have to change the nutritional composition of the foods you eat. You will have to cut down on total calories – that's absolutely basic to weight loss. More important, however, is reducing the percentage of total calories you are getting from fat.

That's how you'll avoid starvation panic in your system. At the same time, you reduce the amount of fat in your food, replacing it with safe, low calorie, nutrient-rich plant foods. This will convince your brain that your body is getting all the nutrition it needs.

In fact, you'll be able to eat more food and feel more satisfied while consuming fewer calories and fats.

Plant foods break down slowly in your stomach, making you feel full longer, and they are rich in vitamins, minerals, trace elements, carbohydrates and protein for energy and muscle-building. This allows your body to burn off its excess stored fat.

CHAPTER 4- WHICH FOODS BURN FAT

Each one of the following foods is clinically proven to promote weight loss. These foods go a step beyond simply adding no fat to your system – they possess special properties that add zip to your system and help your body melt away unhealthy pounds. These incredible foods can suppress your appetite for junk food and keep your body running smoothly with clean fuel and efficient energy.

You can include these foods in any sensible weight-loss plan. They give your body the extra metabolic kick that it needs to shave off weight quickly.

A sensible weight loss plan calls for no fewer that 1,200 calories per day. But Dr. Charles Klein recommends consuming more that that, if you can believe it – 1,500 to 1,800 calories per day. He says you will still lose weight quite effectively at that intake level without endangering your health.

Hunger is satisfied more completely by filling the stomach. Ounce for ounce, the foods listed below accomplish that better than any others. At the same time, they're rich in nutrients and possess special fat-melting talents.

Apples

These marvels of nature deserve their reputation for keeping the doctor away when you eat one a day. And now, it seems, they can help you melt the fat away, too.

First of all, they elevate your blood glucose (sugar) levels in a safe, gentle manner and keep them up longer than most foods.

The practical effect of this is to leave you feeling satisfied longer, say researchers.

Secondly, they're one of the richest sources of soluble fiber in the supermarket. This type of fiber prevents hunger pangs by guarding against dangerous swings or drops in your blood sugar level, says Dr. James Anderson of the University of Kentucky's School of Medicine.

An average size apple provides only 81 calories and has no sodium, saturated fat or cholesterol. You'll also get the added health benefits of lowering the level of cholesterol already in your blood as well as lowering your blood pressure.

Whole Grain Bread

You needn't dread bread. It's the butter, margarine or cream cheese you put on it that's fattening, not the bread itself. We'll say this as often as needed – fat is fattening. If you don't believe that, ponder this – a gram of carbohydrate has four calories, a gram of protein four, and a gram of fat nine. So which of these is really fattening?

Bread, a natural source of fiber and complex carbohydrates, is okay for dieting. Norwegian scientist Dr. Bjarne Jacobsen found that people who eat less than two slices of bread daily weigh about 11 pounds more that those who eat a lot of bread.

Studies at Michigan State University show some breads actually reduce the appetite. Researchers compared white bread to dark, high-fiber bread and found that students who ate 12 slices a day of the dark, high-fiber bread felt less hunger on a daily basis and lost five pounds in two months. Others who ate white bread were hungrier, ate more fattening foods and lost no weight during this time.

So the key is eating dark, rich, high-fiber breads such as pumpernickel, whole wheat, mixed grain, oatmeal and others. The average slice of whole grain bread contains only 60 to 70 calories, is rich in complex carbohydrates – the best, steadiest fuel you can give your body – and delivers surprising amount of protein.

Coffee

Easy does it is the password here. We've all heard about potential dangers of caffeine – including anxiety and insomnia – so moderation is the key.

The caffeine in coffee can speed up the metabolism. In nutritional circles, it's known as a metabolic enhancer, according to Dr. Judith Stern of the University of California at Davis.

This makes sense, since caffeine is a stimulant. Studies show it can help you burn more calories than normal, perhaps up to 10 percent more. For safety's sake, it's best to limit your intake to a single cup in the morning and one in the afternoon. Add only skim milk to tit and try doing without sugar – many people learn to love it that way.

Grapefruit

There's good reason for this traditional diet food to be a regular part of your diet. It helps dissolve fat and cholesterol, according to Dr. James Cerd of the University of Florida. An average sized grapefruit has 74 calories, delivers a whopping 15 grams of pectin (the special fiber linked to lowering cholesterol and fat), is high in vitamin C and potassium and is free of fat and sodium.

It's rich in natural galacturonic acid, which adds to its potency as a fat and cholesterol fighter. The additional benefit here is assistance in the battle against atherosclerosis (hardening of the arteries) and the development of heart disease. Try sprinkling it with cinnamon rather than sugar to take away some of the tart taste.

Mustard

Try the hot, spicy kind you find in Asian import stores, specialty shops and exotic groceries. Dr. Jaya Henry of Oxford Polytechnic Institute in England, found that the amount of hot mustard normally called for in Mexican, Indian and Asian recipes, about one teaspoon, temporarily speeds up the metabolism, just as caffeine and the drug ephedrine do.

"But mustard is natural and totally safe," Henry says. "It can be used every day, and it really works. I was shocked to discover it can speed up the metabolism by as much as 20 to 25 percent for several hours." This can result in the body burning an extra 45 calories for every 700 consumed, Dr. Henry says.

Peppers

Hot, spicy chili peppers fall into the same category as hot mustard, Henry says. He studied them under the same circumstances as the mustard and they worked just as well. A mere three grams of chili peppers were added to a meal consisting of 766 total calories. The peppers' metabolism-raising properties worked like a charm, leading to what Henry calls a diet-induced thermic effect. It doesn't take much to create the effect. Most salsa recipes call for four to eight chilies – that's not a lot.

Peppers are astonishingly rich in vitamins A and C, abundant in calcium, phosphorus, iron and magnesium, high in fiber, free of fat, low in sodium and have just 24 calories per cup.

Potatoes

We've got to be kidding, right? Wrong. Potatoes have developed the same "fattening" rap as bread, and it's unfair. Dr. John McDougal, director of the nutritional medicine clinic at St. Helena Hospital in Deer Park, California, says, "An excellent food with which to achieve rapid weight loss is the potato, at 0.6 calories per gram or about 85 calories per potato." A great source of fiber and potassium, they lower cholesterol and protect against strokes and heart disease.

Preparation and toppings are crucial. Steer clear of butter, milk and sour cream, or you'll blow it. Opt for yogurt instead.

Rice

An entire weight-loss plan, simple called the Rice Diet, was developed by Dr. William Kempner at Duke University in Durham, North Carolina. The diet, dating to the 1930's, makes rice the staple of your food intake. Later on, you gradually mix in various fruits and vegetables.

It produces stunning weight loss and medical results. The diet has been shown to reverse and cure kidney ailments and high blood pressure.

A cup of cooked rice (150 grams) contains about 178 calories — approximately one-third the number of calories found in an equivalent amount of beef or cheese. And remember, whole grain rice is much better for you than white rice.

Soups

Soup is good for you! Maybe not the canned varieties from the store — but old-fashioned, homemade soup promotes weight loss. A study by Dr. John Foreyt of Baylor College of Medicine in Houston, Texas, found that dieters who ate a bowl of soup before lunch and dinner lost more weight than dieters who didn't. In fact, the more soup they ate, the more weight they lost. And soup eaters tend to keep the weight off longer.

Naturally, the type of soup you eat makes a difference. Cream soups or those made of beef or pork are not your best bets. But here's a great recipe:

Slice three large onions, three carrots, four stalks of celery, one zucchini and one yellow squash. Place in a kettle. Add three cans crushed tomatoes, two packets low-sodium chicken bouillon, three cans water and one cup white wine (optional). Add tarragon, basil, oregano, and thyme and garlic powder. Boil, and then simmer for an hour. Serves six.

Spinach

Popeye really knew what he was talking about, according to Dr. Richard Shekelle, an epidemiologist at the University of Texas. Spinach has the ability to lower cholesterol, rev up the metabolism and burn away fat. Rich in iron, beta carotene and vitamins C and E, it supplies most of the nutrients you need.

Tofu

You just can't say enough about this health food from Asia. Also called soybean curd, it's basically tasteless, so any spice or flavoring you add blends with it nicely. A 2½ " square has 86 calories and nine grams of protein. (Experts suggest an intake of about 40 grams per day.) Tofu contains calcium and iron, almost no sodium and not a bit of saturated fat. It makes your metabolism run on high and even lowers cholesterol. With different varieties available, the firmer tofus are goof for stir-frying or adding to soups and sauces while the softer ones are good for mashing, chopping and adding to salads.

CHAPTER 5- OTHER FOODS THAT CAN HELP BURN FAT

It would be unrealistic to think you could successfully lose weight and enjoy what you're eating with a mere handful of foods, no matter how delicious, nutritious and satisfying they may be. So we're going to add an extra roster of fat-fighting foods you can eat along with the great foods mentioned in the last section.

They'll lend different tastes and textures to every meal and provide a wide range of vitamins, minerals, proteins and other vital nutrients. Naturally, each one is high in fiber, low in fat and safe when it comes to sodium content, too.

Many have crunchiness and flavor we've come to desire in snack and nibbling foods. If you're like most of us, you may have a real junk food snacking habit – a habit you're going to have to change in order to slim down. Many of the foods in this section may be worthy substitutes.

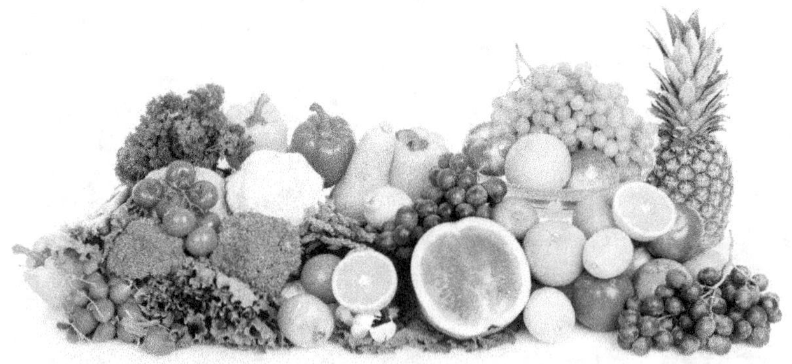

Desiree Osunak
Barley

This filling grain stacks up favorably to rice and potatoes. It has 170 calories per cooked cup, respectable levels of protein and fiber and relatively low fat. Roman gladiators ate this grain regularly for strength and actually complained when they had to eat meat.

Studies at the University of Wisconsin show that barley effectively lowers cholesterol by up to 15 percent and has powerful anti-cancer agents. Israeli scientists say it cures constipation better than laxatives - and that can promote weight loss, too.

Use it as a substitute for rice in salads, pilaf or stuffing, or add to soups and stews. You can also mix it with rice for an interesting texture. Ground into flour, it makes excellent breads and muffins.

Beans

Beans are one of the best sources of plant protein. Peas, beans and chickpeas are collectively known as legumes. Most common beans have 215 calories per cooked cup (lima beans go up to 260). They have the most protein with the least fat of any food, and they're high in potassium but low in sodium.

Plant protein is incomplete, which means that you need to add something to make it complete. Combine beans with a whole grain – rice, barley, wheat, corn – to provide the amino acids necessary to form a complete protein. Then you get the same top-quality protein as in meat with just a fraction of the fat.

Studies at the University of Kentucky and in the Netherlands show that eating beans regularly can lower cholesterol levels.

The most common complaint about beans is that they cause gas. Here's how to contain that problem, according to the U.S. Department of Agriculture (USDA): Before cooking, rinse the beans and remove foreign particles, put in a kettle and cover with boiling water, soak for four hours or longer, remove any beans that float to the top, and then cook the beans in fresh water.

Berries

This is the perfect weight-loss food. Berries have natural fructose sugar that satisfies your longing for sweets and enough fiber so you absorb fewer calories that you eat. British researchers found that the high content of insoluble fiber in fruits, vegetables and whole grains reduces the absorption of calories from foods enough to promote width loss without hampering nutrition.

Berries are a great source of potassium that can assist you in blood pressure control. Blackberries have 74 calories per cup, blueberries 81, raspberries 60 and strawberries 45. So use your imagination and enjoy the berry of your choice.

Broccoli

Broccoli is America's favorite vegetable, according to a recent poll. No wonder. A cup of cooked broccoli has a mere 44 calories. It delivers a staggering nutritional payload and is considered the number one cancer-fighting vegetable. It has no fat, loads of fiber, cancer fighting chemicals called indoles, carotene, 21 times the RDA of vitamin C and calcium.

When you're buying broccoli, pay attention to the color. The tiny florets should be rich green and free of yellowing. Stems should be firm.

Buckwheat

It's great for pancakes, breads, cereal, soups or alone as a grain dish commonly called kasha. It has 155 calories per cooked cup. Research at the All India Institute of Medical Sciences shows diets including buckwheat lead to excellent blood sugar regulation, resistance to diabetes and lowered cholesterol levels. You cook buckwheat the same way you would rice or barley. Bring two to three cups of water to a boil, add the grain, cover the pan, turn down the heat and simmer for 20 minutes or until the water is absorbed.

Cabbage

This Eastern Europe staple is a true wonder food. There are only 33 calories in a cup of cooked shredded cabbage, and it retains all its nutritional goodness no matter how long you cook it. Eating cabbage raw (18 calories per shredded cup), cooked, as sauerkraut (27 calories per drained cup) or coleslaw (calories depend on dressing) only once a week is enough to protect against colon cancer. And it may be a longevity-enhancing food. Surveys in the United States, Greece and Japan show that people who eat a lot of it have the least colon cancer and the lowest death rates overall.

Carrots

What list of health-promoting, fat-fighting foods would be complete without Bugs Bunny's favorite? A medium-sized carrot carries about 55 calories and is a nutritional powerhouse. The orange color comes from beta carotene, a powerful cancer-preventing nutrient (provitamin A).

Chop and toss them with pasta, grate them into rice or add them to a stir-fry. Combine them with parsnips, oranges, raisins, lemon juice, chicken, potatoes, broccoli or lamb to create flavorful dishes. Spice them with tarragon, dill, cinnamon or nutmeg. Add finely chopped carrots to soups and spaghetti sauce — they impart a natural sweetness without adding sugar.

Chicken

White meat contains 245 calories per four ounce serving and dark meat, 285. It's an excellent source of protein, iron, niacin and zinc. Skinned chicken is healthiest, but most experts recommend waiting until after cooking to remove it because the skin keeps the meat moist during cooking.

Corn

It's really a grain — not a vegetable — and is another food that's gotten a bum rap. People think it has little to offer nutritionally and that just isn't so. There are 178 calories in a cup of cooked kernels. It contains good amounts of iron, zinc and potassium, and University of Nebraska researchers say it delivers a high-quality of protein, too.

The Tarahumara Indians of Mexico eat corn, beans and hardly anything else. Virgil Brown, M.D., of Mount Sinai School of Medicine in New York, points out that high blood cholesterol and cardiovascular heart disease are almost nonexistent among them.

Cottage Cheese

As long as we're talking about losing weight and fat-fighting foods, we had to mention cottage cheese.

Low-fat (2%) cottage cheese has 205 calories per cup and is admirably low in fat, while providing respectable amounts of calcium and the B vitamin riboflavin. Season with spices such a dill, or garden fresh vegetable such a scallions and chives for extra zip.

To make it sweeter, add raisins or one of the fruit spreads with no sugar added. You can also use cottage cheese in cooking, baking, fillings and dips where you would otherwise use sour cream or cream cheese.

Figs

Fiber-rich figs are low in calories at 37 per medium (2.25" diameter) raw fig and 48 per dried fig. A recent study by the USDA demonstrated that they contribute to a feeling of fullness and prevent overeating. Subjects actually complained of being asked to eat too much food when fed a diet containing more figs than a similar diet with an identical number of calories.

Serve them with other fruits and cheeses. Or poach them in fruit juice and serve them warm or cold. You can stuff them with mild white cheese or puree them to use as a filling for cookies and low- calorie pastries.

Fish

The health benefits of fish are greater than experts imagined – and they've always considered it a health food.

The calorie count in the average four-ounce serving of a deep-sea fish runs from a low of 90 calories in abalone to a high of 236 in herring. Water-packed tuna, for example, has 154 calories. It's hard to gain weight eating seafood.

As far back as 1985, articles in the New England Journal of Medicine showed a clear link between eating fish regularly and lower rates of heart disease. The reason is that oils in fish thin the blood, reduce blood pressure and lower cholesterol.

Dr. Joel Kremer, at Albany Medical College in New York, discovered that daily supplements of fish oil brought dramatic relief to the inflammation and stiff joints of rheumatoid arthritis.

Greens

We're talking collard, chicory, beet, kale, mustard, Swiss chard and turnip greens. They all belong to the same family as spinach, and that's one of the super-stars. No matter how hard you try, you can't load a cup of plain cooked greens with any more than 50 calories.

They're full of fiber, loaded with vitamins A and C, and free of fat. You can use them in salads, soups, casseroles or any dish where you would normally use spinach.

Kiwi

This New Zealand native is a sweet treat at only 46 calories per fruit. Chinese public health officials praise the tasty fruit for its high vitamin C content and potassium. It stores easily in the refrigerator for up to a month. Most people like it peeled, but the fuzzy skin is also edible.

Leeks

These members of the onion family look like giant scallions, and are every bit as healthful and flavorful as their better-known cousins. They come as close to calorie-free as it gets at a mere 32 calories per cooked cup.

You can poach or broil halved leeks and then marinate them in vinaigrette or season with Romano cheese, fine mustard or herbs. They also make a good soup.

Lettuce

People think lettuce is nutritionally worthless, but nothing could be farther from the truth. You can't leave it out of your weight-loss plans, not at 10 calories per cup of raw romaine. It provides a lot of filling bulk for so few calories. And it's full of vitamin C, too. Go beyond iceberg lettuce with Boston, bibb and cos varieties or try watercress, arugula, radicchio, dandelion greens, purslane and even parsley to liven up your salads.

Melons

Now, here's great taste and great nutrition in a low-calorie package! One cup of cantaloupe balls has 62 calories, on cup of casaba balls has 44 calories, one cup of honeydew balls has 62 calories and one cup of watermelon balls has 49 calories. They have some of the highest fiber content of any food and are delicious. Throw in handsome quantities of vitamins A and C plus a whopping 547 mgs of potassium in that cup of cantaloupe, and you have a fat-burning health food beyond compare.

Oats

A cup of oatmeal or oat bran has only 110 calories. And oats help you lose weight. Subjects in Dr. James Anderson's landmark 12-year study at the University of Kentucky lost three pounds in two months simply by adding 100 grams (3.5 ounces) of oat bran to their daily food intake and nothing else. Just don't expect oats alone to perform miracles – you have to eat a balanced diet for total health.

Onions

Flavorful, aromatic, inexpensive and low in calories, onions deserve a regular place in your diet. One cup of chopped raw onions has only 60 calories, and one raw medium onion (2.15" diameter) has just 42.

They control cholesterol, thin the blood, protect against cholesterol and may have some value in counteracting allergic reactions. Most of all, onions taste good and they're good for you.

Partially boil, peel and bake, basting with olive oil and lemon juice. Or sauté them in white wine and basil, then spread over pizza. Or roast them in sherry and serve over paste.

Pasta

The Italians had it right all along. A cup of cooked paste (without a heavy sauce) has only 155 calories and fits the description of a perfect starch-centered staple. Analysis at the American

Institute of Baking shows pasta is rich in six minerals, including manganese, iron, phosphorus, copper, magnesium and zinc. Also be sure to consider whole wheat pastas, which are even healthier.

Sweet Potatoes

You can make a meal out of them and not worry about gaining a pound – and you sure won't walk away from the table feeling hungry. Each sweet potato has about 103 calories. Their creamy orange flesh is one of the best sources of vitamin A you can consume.

You can bake steam or microwave them. Or add them to casseroles, soups and many other dishes. Flavor with lemon juice or vegetable broth instead of butter.

Tomatoes

A medium tomato (2.5" diameter) has only about 25 calories. These garden delights are low in fat and sodium, high in potassium and rich in fiber.

A survey at Harvard Medical School found that the chances of dying of cancer are lowest among people who eat tomatoes (or strawberries) every week.

And don't overlook canned crushed, peeled, whole or stewed tomatoes. They make sauces, casseroles and soups taste great while retaining their nutritional goodness and low-calorie status. Even plain old spaghetti sauce is a fat-burning bargain when served over pasta, so think about introducing tomatoes into your diet

Turkey

Give thanks to those pilgrims for starting the wonderful tradition of Thanksgiving turkey. It just so happens that this health food disguised as meat is good year-round for weight control.

A four-ounce serving of roasted white meat turkey has 177 calories and dark meat has 211.

Sadly, many folks are still unaware of the versatility and flavor of ground turkey. Anything hamburger can do, ground turkey can do at least as well, from conventional burgers to spaghetti sauce to meat loaf.

Some ground turkey contains skin which slightly increases the fat content. If you want to keep it really lean, opt for ground breast meat. But since this has no added fat, you'll need to add filler to make burgers or meat loaf hold together.

Four ounces of ground turkey has approximately 170 calories and nine grams of fat – about what you'd find in 2.5 teaspoons of butter or margarine. Incredibly, the same amount of regular ground beef (21% fat) has 298 calories and 23 grams of fat.

Buying turkey has become easy. It's no longer necessary to buy a whole bird unless you want to. Ground turkey is available fresh or frozen, as are individual parts of the bird, including drumsticks, thighs, breasts and cutlets.

Yogurt

The non-fat variety of plain yogurt has 120 calories per cup and low-fat, 144. It delivers a lot of protein and , like any dairy food, is rich in calcium and contains zinc and riboflavin.

Yogurt is handy as a breakfast food – cut a banana into it and add the cereal of your choice.

You can find ways to use it in other types of cooking, to – sauces, soups, dips, toppings, stuffing and spreads. Many kitchen gadget departments even sell a simple funnel for making yogurt cheese.

Yogurt can replace heavy creams and whole milk in a wide range of dishes, saving scads of fat and calories.

You can substitute half or all of the higher fat ingredients. Be creative. For example, combine yogurt, garlic powder, lemon juice, a dash of pepper and Worcestershire sauce and use it to top a baked potato instead of piling on fat-laden sour cream.

Desiree Osunak
Supermarkets and health food stores sell a variety of yogurts, many with added fruit and sugar. To control calories and fat content, buy plain non-fat yogurt and add fruit yourself. Apple butter or fruit spreads with little or no added sugar are an excellent way to turn plain yogurt into a delectable sweet treat.

CHAPTER 6-THE BENEFITS OF LOW INTENSITY WORKOUTS

Myth: you'll burn off more fat if you work out at lower intensities versus higher intensities during cardiovascular activities.

Reality: all right, this is technically true, but you have to look at the total picture to comprehend why this would really work against you if you're attempting to slim down.

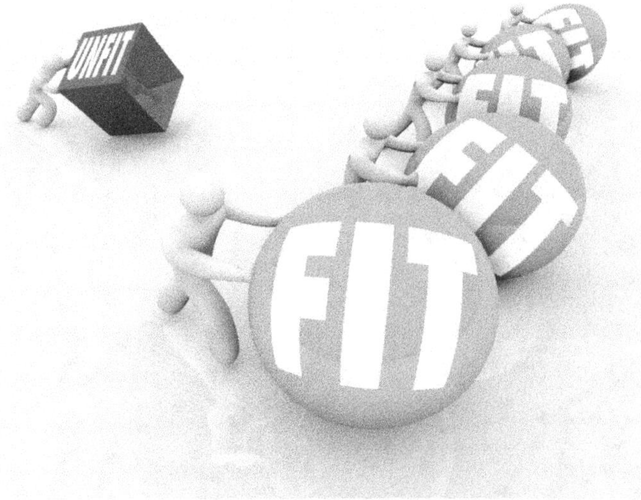

Choose Wisely

This info that I'm going to share with you is based on scientific research and is instructed in every exercise physiology college course.

If you're working out at a low intensity, say 50-60% of your maximum pulse, we're probably safe to say that more than one-half of the calories you're burning off come from fat (let's suppose 60%), and the remainder (approximately 40%) come from sugar, or carbs, in your bloodstream and in your muscles. Bottom line, you burn a greater share of fat at this intensity level than carbs.)

In case you aren't acquainted with intensity based on pulse, 50-60% of your maximum pulse is an easy pace, something you likely could sustain for a long time, perhaps hours.

When you're exercising at greater intensities (suppose 70%-80%), we're safe to state that most individuals are burning off a higher percentage of carbs than fat. Now, simply from this info alone, it may be easy for individuals to believe they're burning more fat at the lower intensities, correct?

The percentages are sure enough greater at the lower intensities. So you may see why so many individuals thought this was the better way to burn fat.

Well, let's have a closer look at what is truly occurring. Let's suppose you've a choice to work out at lower or higher intensity, and let's presume two additional things: 1) among your fitness goals is to drop off body fat and 2) you've a particular amount of time to do your aerobic training; for the sake of this illustration, let's suppose you only have a half-hour. Let's utilize a real world example. We'll call her Joan. One day, Joan works out at 60% (low intensity) of her maximum pulse on the treadmill and she burns off 150 calories. If we may safely say she's burning about 60% of her calories from fat, then she burned off about 90 of those calories from her fat stores. And, if the other 40% of calories burned off came from carbs, then she burned 60 calories from carbs.

The following day, Joan does a higher intensity (80% max pulse) exercise on the treadmill (you have to compare utilizing the same mode of exercise), and she burns 310 calories in a half-hour. If 40% of those calories hailed from fat and 60% from carbs, then she burned 124 calories of fat, and that leaves 186 from carbs.

So, while Joan burned a greater portion of calories from fat with a lower intensity exercise (60% vs. 40%), her absolute value of calories burned off of fat was better in the higher intensity exercise (124 fat calories) versus the lower intensity exercise (90 fat calories). Do you understand why this is a myth and where it may have come from?

Let me make this truly simple. In terms of dropping off body fat, it is not the absolute number of fat calories that counts as much as the absolute number of calories altogether. To exercise off one pound of body fat you have to burn an additional 3500 calories, whether you accomplish it with low intensity or high intensity. I'm sure you are able to see that if you're a busy individual, it pays to get fitter so that you may burn more calories in less time.

However, there's a crucial point about fat burning and intensity level. It has to do with "time to fatigue". Fatigue may impact how many calories you burn. Let me explain.

When Joan is walking at 111 bpm, or 60% of her maximum pulse, if she had the time, she could continue going and going, for a really long time without getting tired. But when she's moving on the treadmill at 148 bpm (80% of her maximum pulse), after a half-hour, she's dog- tired! She's very little energy left. She wasn't fit enough to do that.

Let me explain how fat and carbs get into play here. When you're chiefly utilizing fat as an energy source, as in the case of Joan exercising at 111 bpm, a lower intensity for her, your body may continue to manufacture energy without running out of it. Put differently, it will take a while to tire. However, when you work out at greater intensities, you utilize a bigger percentage of carbs. As the percentage of carbs increases, the sooner you'll tire.

Why is this crucial? I want you to fully comprehend how fat and carbs play a role in exercise and weight loss. Firstly, fats and carbs are equally crucial as energy sources when it comes to exercise.

Secondly, one supplies slow, long-term energy (fat) and the other supplies quick and powerful energy (carbs). Intensity of work out impacts which energy source will prevail over the other.

Thirdly, your intensity level ought to be based on your goals. If your goal is to burn off as many calories as possible in the quickest amount of time, you need to exercise closer to the top end of your capacity.

If your goal is to exercise for a lengthy time period and optimize the number of calories you burn, you'll need to pace yourself. If you merely wish the health benefits, you need to accumulate half-hour a day of activity, which may include exercise and general activity.

Note that the better way to avoid burn out but sustain high levels of fitness and calorie burn is to use interval training, interchanging short bursts of higher intensity training with longer periods of lower intensity training.

Finally, don't forget that the first goal of any exercise program is consistency. It's crucial to begin at your current fitness level and slowly progress in little increments.

CHAPTER 7- DO WE BURN FAT DURING SLEEP?

You don't have to fess up, but how many times have you tested some burn-fat-while-sleeping merchandise? It's understandable why you'd do so. It appears simple, it doesn't require any time, and it appears to work for famous persons! As we talked about earlier, at lower levels of activity, or no activity in the least, we're predominantly utilizing fat as our fuel. As a matter of fact, you're burning fat right now while reading this book (you are able to thank me later...). When you sleep, you're likewise burning off fat.

As a matter of fact, researchers have now discovered a link between the length of sleep you get every night and your weight. In one field of study, over 68,000 ladies were asked to describe how much sleep they got as a rule every night. For sixteen years, the research workers tracked the participants' weight. Final results demonstrate that ladies who got 5 to 6 hours of sleep a night gained more weight than those who slept at least 7 hours every night. One researcher, stated, "Short rest duration is an independent predictor of later weight gain and incident obesity".

In a different study, both gentlemen and ladies were queried about their rest patterns. They discovered that those who got 7 to 8 hours a night were thinner than those who slept 5 to 6 hours. They likewise discovered that those who got less sleep likewise had lower levels of leptin, a hormone that plays a role in body fat and appetite. It's believed that these individuals might be leptin resistant, and consequently they don't get the appetite-suppressing result from it. Now, what if you could you burn off more fat while you rest? You may accomplish this by increasing your metabolism. I understand, easier said than done. It calls for work and patience for this to occur. And, if you slim down, your metabolism really drops as your body has less weight to carry around. All the same, there's a way around this. The way to supercharge metabolism is to increase the total of muscle you have on your body. Now don't panic about becoming bulky or looking like those ladies in the muscle building magazines. They get that way through a lot of hours daily at the gym, a really stern diet, and occasionally a little help from a few banned substances. Most ladies could never look like that, even the ones who wish to.

So, to step-up the amount of muscle you have, you have to integrate strength training. The crucial thing to remember is that for each pound of muscle you have on your body, you'll burn around thirty- five to fifty extra calories a day. This number is deliberated inside the exercise physiology world, but each pound of fat you have will burn off only two calories a day. So whatever number of calories it truly is that muscle burns, it will be entirely more than fat. If you're active and utilizing your muscles (during exercise, for instance) you'll burn off even more calories per pound during the activity.

And so the bottom line here is that in order to burn more fat while you sleep and all throughout the day, you have to strength train to better muscle and your metabolism. Next time you discover a commercial for the new metabolism increaser, spend your cash on some dumbbells alternatively.

CHAPTER 8- THE BEST TIME TO EXERCISE

As you are able to imagine, there has been far-reaching research on this subject. A few of the research studies recommend that we work out in the mid-afternoon for the most beneficial results. There are a lot of reasons for this, but one is that this time of day falls under the correct time based on our innate biorhythms.

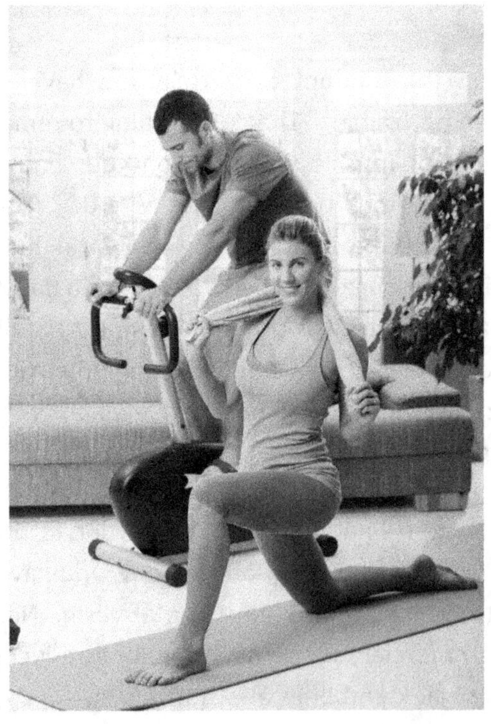

So that's great, let's all go exercise at 2pm each day! Perhaps these researchers may take the time to work out at 2pm, but most individuals I know can't. They have occupations, or they have to fit in workouts around their children's agenda, and a lot of additional reasons.

Desiree Osunak

I don't know who began the idea that it's better to exercise in the morning. Wherever it came from, I've seen this recommendation a lot of times. I read once that you'll burn more fat in the morning as long as you don't consume anything before exercising. There's no way that's going to work for me! For one thing, I have to eat something before I exercise; it's simply the way I am. Second, I'm not a morning individual. It takes a few hours for me to maneuver at full power. If I work out at this time, I really end up burning less calories and I don't get my pulse to the intensity I wish. I'm not burning off much fat this way! It's a big waste of time.

By trial and error, I've found that 10am is the most beneficial time for me to work out. Luckily, I have the sort of schedule that I may fit it in at that time. If I worked regular hours at an office, I'd exercise at lunch, as that was the closest to my ideal time.

So one matter to think about when attempting to ascertain the most beneficial time for you to work out is what time of day you feel your finest. A different way is to determine what time of day you'll really follow through with your work out.

A lot of individuals discover they need to exercise first thing in the morning as if they hold off, the whole day will go by and they'll find excuses for not working out. Others like to work out when they get home to work off tension from their jobs.

I recently met someone who had trouble sticking with a work out schedule. This had been an issue for years; she would exercise for about 3 weeks, then it would go to pieces. She liked to work out after work as she has a nerve-racking job. This worked for a while as she was motivated and she had a coach to hold her accountable.

Finally, she found more and more reasons to skip her exercises. She decided to attempt working out in the morning prior to leaving for work. After a few weeks of getting used to it, she discovered that the exercise truly helped her by giving her the energy she required to deal with her job. She ultimately found a schedule that would work for her.

And so the bottom line is, if you limit yourself to working out when the so-called authorities say you ought to, you'll find yet another barrier to taking control of your personal health. Let your body and your life-style dictate the best time for you. Don't fret about burning fat better at one time or another.

CHAPTER 9- GREAT WORKOUT ROUTINES

There are gobs of cardiovascular activities that may help you burn off fat. Cardiovascular activities help you burn off calories, make you more fit, and better your health. Everybody wishes to know which one is the most beneficial for his or her specific goals.

Let's have a look at what cardiovascular activity is first off. Plainly put, cardiovascular exercise is movement that utilizes the major muscle groups of your body in a rhythmical pattern.

When identifying the activity, we utilize duration (how long), intensity level (pulse, rating of perceived effort), frequency (times per week), and mode (sort of activity).

As we talked about earlier, intensity and length are related to one another. You are able to work out longer at lower intensities, but you'll burn off more calories in a shorter time period at a higher intensity.

As for frequency, authorities deviate in their recommendations. The scope tends to be anyplace from 3 to 5 days a week. The last element of cardiovascular activity is mode.

Here are a few modes of cardiovascular action:

- Walking (outdoors or treadmill)
- Running (outdoors or treadmill)
- Swimming
- Rollerblading
- Step climbing

- Elliptical conditioning
- Water aerobic exercise
- Aerobic exercise/step classes
- Biking

There are a lot more! I'm certain you are able to think of a few I didn't include on this list. Which of these actions do you believe will be most effective for slimming down? How about for bringing down cholesterol? Toning your body? Increasing vitality? Most crucial to our discussion, which action is best for burning off fat?

Well, the reality is, it's a trick question-- they're all equally effective. Just like picking out the best time of day for you to exercise, you need to pick the type of cardiovascular activity that you like the most and are most likely to follow. You'll be much more consistent and reap more advantages when your activity is pleasurable.

Let me interject one crucial detail. As you advance through your workouts, you'll have to add and keep assortment in your exercise routine. If you only walk on the treadmill, after some time your body will get used to it and no longer continue to better.

Pick a 2nd activity like rollerblading or biking so your body has to adjust to new activities. This is called cross-training and it's crucial to utilize so your body doesn't get used to one activity. It's likewise crucial so you don't get a repetitive motion injury from exercising only one way.

Consider Your Present Exercise Routine

Do you utilize mostly front to back movements, like running, walking or elliptical training? If so, attempt rollerblading, sliding, or tennis. These actions add a sideways element for variety.

Are you working out inside? Attempt walking or running outside. It's surprising how much tougher it can be to run outdoors when you're used to simply utilizing the treadmill.

Are you only exercising at the gym? Discover an alternate activity you may do at home in case of inclemency or if you just don't feel like getting out.

Are you merely utilizing the bike? Begin walking and add some impact to your workout - your bones will appreciate it! If you're participating in all impact activities, take a look at swimming or bicycling one or two times a week to prevent injury.

The primary point here is that the most effective cardiovascular training is the one you like to do and will do on a steady basis, and don't forget to find a few different activities for cross-training.

CHAPTER 10- WHEN TO EAT

This isn't precisely about burning off fat. But if you're attempting to slim down, I'm certain you have wondered about this. I've heard that you ought to eat following exercise to replace glucose and glycogen supplies. I've likewise been told not to eat following exercise in order to heighten calorie burn. To be truthful, I don't know what you ought to do or shouldn't do. I truly don't think anybody does.

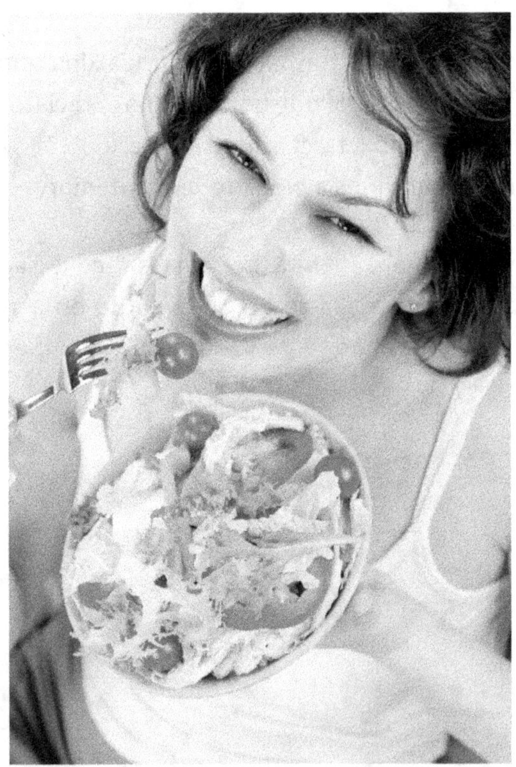

Here is just a little sample of advice from a lot of respected authors and health associations:

Avoid arduous exercise for at least 2 hours following eating a meal.

Wait approximately twenty minutes before eating following exercise.

Eat something light 30 minutes prior to exercising in the morning. Make sure to eat inside 2 hours after to restore fuel to your muscles.

Work out in the morning on an empty stomach.

Consume a low fat, complex-carbohydrate meal or snack one to four hours prior to exercise.

Eat .45 gm of carbs per pound of bodyweight one hour prior to exercise.

Like I stated, I truly don't think anybody knows for certain. In my judgment and experience, everybody is different, you have to experiment with when, and what you ought to eat before and/or following exercise. If you eat prior to exercise and you feel sick to your stomach or sluggish, you likely should cut down on the amount or not eat at all. If you feel dizzy or weak, you might have to eat more or eat closer to working out. If you're hungry following exercise, that's a great indication that you ought to eat! In all cases, make sure to eat when you're hungry and stop when you're full.

The concept of intuitive eating works here, too. If you feed your body established on its physical needs and demands, you'll eventually return to your natural weight. Bottom line, you'll have to experiment with when you eat and the sorts of food you eat to ascertain what is best for your body.

CONCLUSION

In the battle of the bulge and the fight against fat, boosting your metabolism is one of the best weapons you can have in your arsenal. Learn that increasing your metabolism means not starving yourself, it means getting out there and putting on some lean muscle mass, eating small meals throughout the day to keep your blood sugar level and it even means avoiding stress.

Getting your internal fire burning will help you lose weight and feel better about yourself. Who could ask for more?

ABOUT THE AUTHOR

Desiree Osunak has been a fitness strainer for over eight years and she knows that a metabolism that is functioning properly provides the individual with all the energy that they need to get through the day. They will also feel much better as well. A slow metabolism makes the individual feel sluggish and tends to prevent them from doing much.

Desiree has written a book to help persons learn just how important it is to have a metabolism that is working properly. She even outlines the foods that can help to keep the metabolism working properly. Her main aim is to inform and educate as many persons as possible.

www.ingramcontent.com/pod-product-compliance
Lightning Source LLC
Chambersburg PA
CBHW070051260726
48658CB00002B/845